Not in pain (Revised and Updated Second Edition) :

A Novel Approach to Ending Chronic Pain

by

Dr. Kevin J. Bryan

without approval from the publisher or creator.

Table of content

Introduction

The pandemic of pain

Americans' opinions about people suffering are reflected in how they handle their discomfort. From the 1940s through the 1960s, there were more injured veterans, which raised attention on pain and its management. The concept of the person in pain has alternated between being seen as a physiological construct and as an actual person, whose experience of

their agony may be influenced by social, emotional, and cultural variables.

Conceptually, the pain has a medical foundation as well as a political context, varying, for instance, between empirical proof of impairment brought on by pain and irrational fears of malingering. In the 20th century, pharmaceutical pain treatment became the norm. Increased opioid usage resulted from perceptions of undertreatment, first for those experiencing cancer-related pain and then for people experiencing non-cancer pain without the multifaceted care that was planned.

The pharmaceutical industry and the medical community overstated the absence of addiction associated with these drugs when used to treat non-cancer pain; this overstatement was later shown to be untrue and purposefully misleading. The pandemic of opioid prescriptions started in the 1990s. Numerous initiatives have been made to reduce opioid usage, both in cancer patients and cancer survivors as well as in patients with non-cancer diseases, in response to an alarming increase in opioid-related fatalities.

Over 630 000 people in the United States died from drug overdoses between 1999 and 2016; the majority of these drug-related fatalities were brought on by opioids that were prescribed for pain. The first wave of the opioid crisis is thought to have begun between 1999 and 2010 when there was a steady rise in the number of overdose fatalities caused by opioid painkillers. Following this wave, the United States was heavily impacted by the second and third waves of opioid overdose fatalities caused by heroin and illicitly produced fentanyl (IMF), respectively.

Fatalities increased from 52 404 in 2015 to 72 000 (provisional) deaths by 2017. Synthetic opioids (like fentanyl) have recently been urged to be excluded from the categorization of prescription opioid-related fatalities to more accurately describe these deaths as increasingly coming from illegal opioids. This categorization has significant ramifications for the problem-solving approaches that we cover under potential solutions.

The use of opioids has increased over the past 20 years, and this article examines how our understanding of pain has changed over time, as well as how it has affected the political, legal, and regulatory systems in the United States (at first using the disability of World War II veterans as a stand-in for the subjective symptom of pain). Finally, we go through existing ways to combat the opioid problem, including regulations, laws, monitoring, and other measures. An elaboration of the social backdrop is not possible due to space.

Descartes developed the first modern theories of pain in the middle of the 1600s with his notion of pain specificity. A nerve traveled from a painful stimulation on the body's surface via the spinal cord to a location in the brain where pain might be felt. This idea had multiple consequences. The pain was a simple physiologic notion, but the emotional, cultural, or social nuances of the message were ignored, and only one place in the brain processed pain information. Most crucially, in this understanding, the body and the intellect were distinct.

The following three centuries saw an evolution in our understanding of pain as metaphysical explanations and the power of the church diminished, and suffering and psychological factors were further minimized, but by the 1900s, the idea of suffering and the psychological factor was once again accepted. Finally, with the 1968 publication of the Gate Control Theory of Pain, the idea of modulation of the pain message gained greater significance. The continued development of this theory has aided in the reintroduction of aspects of suffering—psychological, spiritual, and cultural—that had been ignored for the previous four centuries. This theory was developed in part as a result of the political and cultural ethos that was already in place and developing concurrently with our understanding of how pain works, from a straightforward transmission along a well-defined pathway to modulation of the message by brain regions that react to related factors like stoicism learned from culture.

With the invention and widespread use of morphine for wounded Civil War troops, pain management techniques started to advance in the United States in the middle of the 19th century. Some doctors and some patients hesitated to use anesthetics and analgesics in the late 1800s and early 1900s, preferring to depend on nonpharmacologic treatments instead. With the return of the wounded World War II troops in the middle of the 1900s, pharmacologic treatment had become the mainstay of rehabilitation, which was partly influenced by the same political and cultural attitude.

Before the widespread use of anesthetic substances like ether and chloroform, whose usage started in the late 1840s, as well as subsequently in wounded soldiers and civilians during the Civil War period, Bourke has documented accounts of intense agony. Former soldiers who continued to take morphine after the war faced a problem. Due to their utilization for continuous chronic pain, morphine and heroin were both subject to limitations in the early 1900s.

Before World War II, little use was made of veteran services.

Both anesthesiologists Henry Beecher and John Bonica documented how troops with serious and sometimes fatal wounds suppressed their agony and concentrated on getting back to their combat colleagues. Barbiturates, which were administered to others who were clearly in agony, helped them feel better. These findings resulted in a fresh recognition of the importance of social, cultural, and psychological (such as bonding on the battlefield) elements.

A huge increase in the number of wounded veterans and the demand for assistance for them resulted from the suffering that veterans continued to experience after sustaining their injuries during combat and after returning to civilian life in the US. Wailoo explores the role politics, both governmental and medical, played in the treatment of chronic pain and disability as its proxy in the late 1940s and 1950s.

Others who fought to trust the person, like Beecher and Bonica, when the handicap was brought on by the subjective symptom of pain, were up against those who sought to quantify the issue for either monetary recompense or to deny the issue even existed. Veterans of World Wars I, II, and the Korean War combined to increase the number of disabled people from 0.5 million in 1940 to 3 million by 1960, which is significant in understanding the development of the present pandemic.

The cost of medications is not the root of this worldwide epidemic of avoidable pain; oral morphine may be produced for pennies per dosage. However, the International Narcotics Control Board reports that the use of opioids is "insufficient" or "extremely inadequate" to address basic medical requirements in over 121 nations. If they get prevalent illnesses including cancer, cardiovascular disease, HIV, chronic lung disease, and diabetes, an estimated 83 percent of the world's population will experience significant discomfort.

States have a dual responsibility to safeguard the availability of opioid medications for medical use and to safeguard people against misuse and reliance on them. Many nations give the latter an excessive amount of weight at the cost of the former.

Many patients are unable to get necessary medications like oral morphine and other efficient analgesics as a consequence of such uneven regulations.

They could be incorrectly deemed ineligible, they might need a specialist visit, and even if they had a prescription, they would only be able to get a few days' worths of morphine, which they would have to ask for in person. Other problems include a lack of training for medical professionals in the use of painkillers, patients' reservations about using them, and physicians' fear of being held accountable for prescribing them because of too harsh rules.

But patients do not have to endure discomfort till they pass away. Patricia had advanced cervical cancer and was hospitalized in November 2013. She was moved to the hospital's palliative care department in March 2016, where she now takes morphine to aid with pain management. She is now pain-frcc for the first time while worrying about caring for her aging parents. She would not have gotten this kind of care in Mexico only two years ago since the restrictions were so onerous that the majority of physicians simply did not prescribe these drugs, and very few pharmacies had them on hand.

But Mexico has lately made significant advancements.

According to a Mexican palliative care expert, access to opioids has never been easy in Mexico. Only anesthesiologists and pain doctors who were ready to fulfill the high criteria of the Regulatory Authority were allowed to administer morphine and other strong opioids. The new rules have led to a rise in the number of doctors who are authorized to write heavy opioid prescriptions, an increase in the number of pharmacies carrying morphine, and an improvement in the accessibility of opioids for pain sufferers.

On the opposite side of the globe, in India, the Parliament of India approved legislation in 2013–2014 that simplified federal and state laws governing restricted substances. However, as in many other nations, individual states must put these simplified rules into practice. More importantly, professional organizations must include palliative care training in undergraduate medical and nursing curricula if India's 1.25 billion people are to have access to pain relief and palliative care.

WHO is offering support globally as the epidemic of unnecessary pain persists. According to Gilles Forte, WHO's Coordinator for Policy Access and Use, "WHO put morphine on its first Essential Medicines List in 1977 and deems it the gold standard in pain treatment and alleviation." Every nation should put morphine on its list of fundamental medications and guarantee that it is always available in medical institutions.

Access to painkillers will be improved via other WHO initiatives.

Clinical treatment recommendations for cancer pain are now being revised, and advice has been offered on how to ensure balance in national policy on banned substances. Additionally, WHO collaborates with nations to determine the conditions for enhancing access to opioid analgesics. These initiatives will support, among other things, the creation of services that may aid in the eradication of the pandemic of avoidable suffering.

Chapter 1

Pain Cycle

An injury that makes it difficult for your body to move normally might result in chronic discomfort.

An injury that makes it difficult for your body to move normally might result in chronic discomfort. The major effects of the pain cycle are imbalanced movements that result in bad posture. By examining this cycle, we can observe how your body responds to pain brought on by an injury and how it might lead to a chain reaction of perilous occurrences with permanent consequences.

The Pain Cycle is a graphic tool that aids patients in understanding how pain may negatively and self-reinforcingly influence many elements of their lives.

The Self-Care Cycle, a companion figure, illustrates the benefits of using a variety of self-management techniques to reduce or eliminate the effects of pain.

What Sets Off the Pain Cycle?

An injury sets off the agony cycle. A person must alter how he or she stands, moves, or rests as a result of this injury.

The body's tendency to encourage certain activities to prevent pain is what starts the pain cycle. Your body will discover other ways of bending if you have an injury to your arm and it hurts to bend it in a specific manner. Depending on the severity of the injury, a different amount of time may be needed to recuperate. Your body will instinctively try to discover a deformed motion that doesn't hurt when it hurts to move properly.

Effects of the Pain Cycle That Last

Depending on how serious the injury was, the healing period might be lengthy or brief. Some muscles, ligaments, or nerves may have been acclimated to moving in a twisted manner throughout the healing process. Even after the damage has healed, these movements are continually used. The novel motions may result in persistent discomfort. The body developed these movements to mitigate discomfort, but today the motions are the source of suffering.

How Can the Cycle of Pain Be Broken?

Through movements that release your body's aching joints and muscles, you may break the cycle of pain. One organic strategy to break the pain cycle is to restore mobility to the proper posture. It might be stressful to try to promote natural movements when your body still encourages artificial ones. Before attempting any treatments that can be more harmful than helpful, it is advised to see a chronic pain specialist. The proper pain management strategy may guarantee that your body keeps promoting homeostasis.

Chapter 2

Comparing our perception of pain to the reality

We are all intimately acquainted with suffering, yet we don't comprehend what it means objectively. I've seen that a person's mental state, such as when they're hypnotized or anxious, may impact how they feel pain, but we don't know how to interpret this finding. Sometimes people with identical physical ailments describe experiencing pain indistinctly different ways.

It also seems that occasionally situations that did not originally cause pain cause individuals to develop a pain threshold. Is there a range of pain in each of these situations, or might it be that the pain is constant while something else is shifting? How is a query like that answered? Opiate users may claim that even if they are in pain, it does not disturb them. According to some specialists, we should assume that these folks are speaking incorrectly since there is no such thing as pain that is not uncomfortable.

Others utilize the assertions made by opiate-dependent individuals as evidence and inspiration for novel pain theories. Even if their pain behavior resembles that of those whose pain is undeniably genuine, some physicians contend that some persons who feel they are in pain are only imagining it. Others contend that a true report of pain removes any question as to whether or not the patient is indeed experiencing it.

How can we decide which course of action, if any, is appropriate in these situations? Individuals who are suffering as well as the scientific study that would seek remedies for them are impacted by the varied perspectives that people have on these matters. But it seems that if scientists can't agree on when and how much pain is present in their patients, they won't be able to settle these disagreements via empirical research. Scientists may be able to agree on when their subjects are experiencing "pain" and the corresponding physiology by using an arbitrary but precise definition of the phenomenon.

However, it is unable to provide light on the aforementioned problems since they relate to our everyday idea rather than the arbitrary, scientifically defined ones. Some philosophers, such as Dennett, see the aforementioned conflicts as proof that our idea of pain is nonsensical (1978). They contend that there is no concrete evidence to support the claims that pain may be learned, imagined, or experienced by someone and yet not disturb them. This conclusion, in our opinion, is hasty, and we still have much to learn about pain from the challenging issues mentioned above.

"science has to explain that form of experience, not something else wholly unrelated to it," adding that "the common-sense term [pain] does appear to pick out an essential kind of experience - even if common sense only faintly understands the experience."

1, I'll try to clarify a few things, focusing on the idea that suffering must somehow be understood in terms of perception. Additionally, we want to promote the much-needed conversation between philosophers and psychologists on how to use words like "sensation" and "perception.

We end by noting that conceptual analysis can only go so far in helping us understand how pain affects perception and that the ideal cognitive model to use in determining how pain affects perception must be based on empirical evidence. Not a Simple Sensation: Pain The idea that pain is a kind of experience brought on by somatic pain receptors sending signals to a pain center in the brain is one that is sometimes taught in medical textbooks.

This perspective initially assumes that pain is a fundamental sensation, i.e., a straightforward linear process that starts with the activation of sensors at the pain's site and concludes with the determination that there is pain there. This perspective does not seem to acknowledge the complex information surrounding pain as previously mentioned. According to experts who research pain, such a perspective ignores all of the fascinating intricacies that surround pain.

The idea that pain is a fundamental feeling is likewise extensively rejected in the contemporary philosophical literature. Philosophers prefer to draw attention to the fact that there doesn't appear to be a particular kind of feeling that all pains share, among other things. Additionally, it seems that the brain's pain processing region does not receive such sensory impulses. Instead, several brain areas are activated whenever someone experiences pain.

The most promising of these alternative explanations of pain, which include some form of function for the perception of the idea of pain, have proliferated as a result of these discoveries, 1 p. 326 1652. Perception and Pain Most people think of perception as complicated information processing that starts with low-level input from the sense organs and ends with a portrayal of some feature of the external environment. Scientists believe that cognitive characteristics including attention and stability, as well as other sensory modalities, connections, memories, beliefs, and attitudes, have an impact on this processing.

As a result, one's expectations, the object of one's attention, and what one was seeing a second before may all affect what one sees (or does not perceive). What one sees may have an impact on what one hears. Depending on which cuisine one believes is more appropriate for the environment, one may perceive the fragrance of popcorn or rice. Researchers studying pain have shown that if the pain is a perception-based phenomenon, then one may anticipate that such effects would affect how one perceives pain.

One may experience pain even when there is simply a gentle touch and no physical harm, much as one can "see" a deer when shooting only to find out later that they accidentally shot the neighbor's dog. In reality, doctors may more readily resist the urge to label unusual instances of pain as being "merely in the mind" and researchers can attribute the enigmatic nature of all of the empirical evidence discussed above to the intricacies of perception. They may accept the patient's assertion that his pain is genuine if they believe that pain is the product of a perceptual process.

It is now possible to understand pain, which was always thought to be "only in the mind," as a very real result of the head. However, stating that pain has some connection to perception is not all that significant. How does the perception of pain relate to the perceptual process? When we experience pain, what precisely do we perceive? How to Feel Pain Rarely is explicitly stated, but one theory on pain holds that the sensation of pain is the actual sensation of pain. The writing of scientists sometimes gives the impression that pain is the target of a pain-detecting perceptual mechanism.

Chapman (1986) states that "noxious sensory input is characterized by severe ambiguity unless the stimulus source is evident and the stimulus is powerful. The impulse barrage may be classified under unclear conditions at a variety of information processing levels. Such categorization may diminish it to a minimal level of pain, resulting in an experience that is not pain but rather another tangentially related feeling (such as tightness or cramping), or enhance the sensory signal and link it to a serious hazard.

2. Sometimes refers to the experience of pain specifically and refers to it as an instance of "inner perception." We disagree with the idea that pain is a tangible thing that can be perceived. Whatever one means by perception, in our opinion, it must at the very least entail information processing that results in a representation of how something in the world is. 2 P. 162 Whatever pain is, a perceptual system has not developed to be able to detect it in the outside world (or even in the body). We believe that to believe differently would be to take clichés about pain, such as "I have an ache in my shoulder," too seriously.

The sensation of pain is a result of perception. Pain may be a feeling, but it results in a difficult perceptual process. According to Hall (1989), experiencing pain is equivalent to experiencing pain sensations, the latter of which are feelings that are felt when the body is in a certain perceptual condition. One is left wondering exactly what Hall has in mind since he doesn't specify what the objects of such awareness are.

According to his theory, a person may experience the same pain in a pleasurable or terrible way, based on their psychology as well as the possible evolutionary function that a specific kind of pain sensation may have served. In other words, on the one side, there are pain sensations, which are the result of intricate perceptual processes, and on the other, there is the issue of how we feel about those sensations. Looking more broadly at the distinction between perception and sensation may be helpful in better understanding this idea of pain. Unfortunately, philosophers have a lot to say about something that they disagree on.

We might state that sensations are often thought to be non-conceptual in nature and inextricably linked to experience. They are often considered to be non-representative as well. In contrast, perceptions are often thought to be representational, involve conceptual or cognitive components, and are, at least in theory, independent of experience. Let's suppose that, under Peacocke (1983), the representational content of a perception is how it depicts the state of the world. According to some philosophers, perceptions are entirely representational.

Others assert that while they are representational, they also have certain sensational qualities, namely what is left after their representational content has been removed. I believe that seeing Hall's viewpoint on suffering from the second angle will help you better grasp it. For humans to experience pain, some type of perception must exist. When the representational content of this experience is removed, just the feeling is left, and that is what pain is. But it is difficult to fully understand Hall's suggestion without knowing what he has in mind for the aim of this perceptual process.

What exactly is perceived? And why would one assume that the feeling resulting from this perception has nothing to do with the emotive component of our pain experience, which may very well be a representational component of the linked perception? Why, in this perspective, wouldn't the ensuing feeling we name pain to have this emotional component? Hall's theory is debatable since psychologists believe that sensations are low-level stimulations of sensory nerves that send messages linearly to higher-level brain areas without "top-down" impacts.

however, that feelings are a result of perception. This is more than just a case of Hall using incorrect terminology because, if he were to substitute the term "phenomenal experience" for "sensation," he would lose a key element of his theory that distinguishes it from the others: the idea that our overall experience of pain differs from the way the pain itself feels. According to Hall, whether we feel the pain to be unbearably terrible or not at all, it is always the same specific sensation that we are bothered by or not by.

3. Pain is the quality or perception of a perception. An alternate perspective reduces suffering to a specific perceptual event. It is believed that researchers investigating pain are exploring a sophisticated method of perception. Nociceptors, which activate in reaction to stress or tissue injury, generally start the process. The information transmitted from the nociceptive system functions as both a (1) warning system, informing about tissue damage or threat of damage, its extent, and its location, and (2) a reminding system, informing repeatedly that injury is present in a particular area of the body so that physical movement will be adjusted to best facilitate healing. A-delta fibers dominate the warning system, which generates a faster, brighter signal. C-fibers predominate in the rcminder system, which generates a very unpleasant and diffuse signal. It seems logical to suggest that what is being perceived when one experiences pain is the state of the body, and in particular, in cases of injury or impending injury, information about the body at the location where the injury is taking place.

This is because any perceptual system that is to account for pain must be processing signals produced by these two systems. Pitcher (1970) expresses this opinion. He contends that experiencing pain only involves recognizing physical harm. We refer to the condition of perceiving bodily harm as an instance of feeling pain because the condition of misperceiving physical damage is sufficiently comparable to the condition of perceiving bodily damage.

We experience what looks to be physical harm and have "an instantaneous impulse to shift [our]'state of consciousness,' an immediate desire to wish it to cease, just as a person experiencing pain typically does."

4. This may be comparable to situations when we tell the eye doctor that we see spots while being 100% convinced that there are none where we are looking. According to Pitcher, the typical discomfort associated with being in pain is brought on by 3 The contrast between Hall's narrative and the account (Nelkin, 1991).

Nelkin suggests that the perceptual state of pain is non-inferentially appraised. As a result, pain cannot be felt. Instead, there are representational phenomenal states that are appraised right away via a kind of introspection (for example, the feeling in my foot that is analogous to the experience of being cut by a sharp instrument) (i.e., that [sensation in my foot] means bodily damage.) The parallel may highlight how crucial part perception is to Hall's story. 4 Pitcher, p. 385, states that it is uncomfortable for humans to notice physical harm, maybe even always being so.

A significantly different perspective on pain is held by Douglas (1998), who emphasizes that it is a kind of reaction to an item, such as a boil or burn, or a reaction to an event that is often harmful to the body, such as a slap or a stab. In his opinion, when we observe or sense this bodily harm, we experience pain. In other words, pain is a mental process attribute. Douglas, like Pitcher, does not consider pain to be a perception-based, sensation-based, or any other kind of mental object.

Be aware that according to this perspective, if one senses physiological harm (by using the proper perceptual processes), one experiences pain. The experience doesn't need to have a certain characteristic for it to qualify as painful. The fact that you are seeing something in this manner automatically establishes that it has a feeling, and that feeling is pain. At first glance, it seems that pain may theoretically not be troublesome from this perspective. In this context, the instances of opiate-dependent patients might be comprehended.

The drug's action causes the impression of physical harm to have a different, maybe less distressing, nature than usual. Comparisons and Contrasts What would distinguish Douglas's theory that pain is the way something feels to be perceived from Hall's theory that pain is the feeling that results from perception? Given Hall's account's gaps, the answer to this issue must be very hypothetical. However, it seems to go somewhat like this: While not a mental entity in and of itself, Douglas believes that pain is inextricably linked to both our ideas and our emotions.

The way we interpret—read: represent—what is occurring to us and the feelings this interpretation arouses are fundamental to how perception feels. Our impression of physical harm is quite cognitively permeable; our emotions and ideas may affect how painful we feel. In contrast, Hall is quite explicit about his intention to disregard the emotive component of pain perception. Due to the numerous beliefs that affect the perceptual process from which the pain experience is produced, a pain sensation may be of one kind vs another.

However, the experience is ultimately just that—a sensation. For Douglas, the way we experience that anguish is a different thing. Our feelings and the evolution facts have an impact on it. We interpret this to suggest that, although emotional variables may not directly affect the kind of pain that an individual experiences, they may have an impact on how that pain feels for a certain individual. Though the opinions of Hall, Pitcher, and Douglas are logically distinct, from a scientific perspective, it can seem that they are practically equal.

That is, it's possible that each theory makes the same empirical predictions and that every piece of empirical evidence has an explanation. For instance, pain is a result of a perceptual process in each view. From each perspective, alterations in the other factors influencing the perceptual process may have an impact on how painful something feels in addition to nociception being blocked. For instance, by changing the emphasis of a subject's attention away from a physical disorder, his or her perceptual processing may change, which, from all three perspectives, might have a favorable effect on how they perceive their suffering.

Pitcher and Douglas both believe that the subject's impression of physical harm alters as a result of the attention being shifted. Perhaps less serious physical harm is experienced. Pitcher believes that altering one's discomfort is equivalent to altering one's sense of physical injury. According to Douglas, the new impression would feel different from the old one in this instance because it would be less painful. As opposed to these viewpoints, Hall's theory offers two additional possibilities: either this altered perception would result in the experience of brand-new, less unpleasant sensations, or the redirected attention might not affect perception or the derivative pain sensations at all, but rather affect the subject's emotional response to these sensations, making the same pain sensation less unpleasant. Each perspective also provides a means of comprehending pain as a teachable concept (and unlearned). Imagine learning that a substance you often deal with is extremely carcinogenic and then discovering for the first time that breathing it in hurts. Or possibly, after receiving numerous deep muscle massages every week, one starts to believe in their value and stops finding them uncomfortable.

Since beliefs are recognized to affect perception and pain is regarded on all three accounts to be a function of perception, it follows that learning, or gaining new beliefs, may result in new pain experiences or even the removal of pain. Pitcher and Douglas discovered a second approach to learning about pain. According to their theories, changing one's emotional reactions to certain events might result in changing one's beliefs, which, in turn, can change one's perceptions.

Finally, despite it seeming that Hall maintains the idea that pain sensations are unaffected by emotions, it is evident that he would let the fresh emotions that might sometimes accompany new beliefs result in fresh experiences of the same pain sensations. A proponent of Hall may thus claim that under the aforementioned scenarios, a person begins to perceive a certain pain feeling as more or less unpleasant, for example. Note that the painful feelings are consistent on this account. There is just the learned and unlearned experience of a certain feeling; there is no taught (or unlearned) suffering.

We think that how one approaches doing clinically focused pain research might directly depend on how one perceives the connection between pain and perception. One could wonder how each of the aforementioned ideas might approach pain management. Pitcher believed that since pain is defined as the perception of bodily harm, the only way to alleviate pain without treating the affected body part is to alter how that harm is perceived. According to Douglas, the goal could be the same since Douglas believes that pain is a characteristic of perception.

Of course, there would be a variety of methods to influence how physical harm was perceived. One might concentrate on the lower levels of processing or "top-down" factors like beliefs and emotions. Some of these techniques could be compared to instructing a subject to become painless. According to Hall's theory of pain, there are several ways to cure pain, which calls for various study focuses. To alleviate pain, one might try to change how the person perceives his suffering while maintaining the pain itself. This objective would concentrate on his emotional state.

Or, as Pitcher and Douglas would have you do, you may try to alter the feeling by altering the associated perception. But according to Hall, this goal would require influencing higher-level ideas or maybe lower-level processes, but not, it would seem, emotions. On Hall's definition of pain, it is impossible to rule out an alternative potential for pain relief; it is possible that medicine, for example, may affect the feeling that ordinarily underlies a certain experience without changing the impression itself.

This would pave the way for therapies that work to alter the sensations brought on by these perceptions rather than our perceptions or our emotions. Pitcher's comprehension of suffering makes this notion impossible. From Douglas's viewpoint on pain, a similar potential may be present: perhaps a medicine might affect how it feels to have a certain perception. Whether anything other than the perception itself affects how a perception feels would rely on this.

Chapter 3

Our Musculoskeletal Sole: Feet and Ankles

The foot and ankle were created specifically to transfer the weight of the body. The foot may adapt to accommodate a variety of surfaces. The bones, ligaments, and fascia are arranged to form a spring-like arch, and there are thick pads beneath the heels and toes, which collectively serve as shock absorbers.

Numerous arthropathies affect the foot and ankle, and because of the concentrated strains on the joints, there may be additional issues.

Due to their rising prevalence and severe detrimental effects on patients' quality of life, musculoskeletal disorders of the foot and ankle pose a significant public health risk. Patients with musculoskeletal problems of the foot and ankle typically employ non-pharmacological therapy as the first line of treatment. Based on the information that is currently available, this review gives an overview of the evaluations and non-invasive treatment alternatives.

According to my research, people who have foot and ankle discomfort simultaneously experience several alignments, motion, load distribution, and muscle performance limitations, which may be seen during static or dynamic activities. The relationship between the foot and proximal joints is also supported by epidemiological and clinical investigations. For instance, osteoarthritis (OA) and discomfort in the knee and hip have both been associated with abnormal foot anatomy.

Recent developments in plantar load distribution monitoring and motion capture technologies provide prospects for accurate dynamic evaluations of the foot and ankle.

The main goals of therapy are to provide pain relief, restore mechanics (alignment, motion, and/or load distribution), and enable patients with musculoskeletal problems of the foot and ankle to resume their preferred level of activity participation.

A combination therapy that targets both local and general deficits in the foot has shown promising outcomes given that the majority of patients present with multiple impairments. Comprehensive rehabilitation treatments, such as early identification, foot-based therapies (such orthoses), and wellness-based approaches for physical activity and self-management, have proven effective, especially in those with rheumatoid arthritis and other rheumatic disorders.

Few randomized clinical studies have explicitly examined individuals with foot or ankle issues to provide broad insights into this field, despite substantial advancements in the evaluation and treatment of foot and ankle diseases during the last ten years. As a result, the quality and breadth of the research I offer in this review, as well as the current recommendations, differ. The results of this analysis point to the need for more research into the factors that go into musculoskeletal problems of the foot and ankle being assessed and treated.

The burden of foot and ankle ailments will grow as the world's aging population increases, which is a significant public health concern. These disorders are nearly twice as common in people with rheumatoid arthritis (RA) as in the general population. However, rheumatology specialists have only recently begun to pay attention to foot and ankle diseases. Very little research has been done on the foot and non-surgical foot therapies that could help foot pain and accompanying rheumatic disorders, compared to non-invasive adjustments for joint malalignment at the knee and hip.

This review's goal is to provide a summary of the most recent research on diseases affecting the musculoskeletal system of the ankle and foot, with an emphasis on diagnosis and non-pharmacological, non-invasive treatment options. We will discuss the evaluation and management of foot pain and ankle pain individually in the sections that follow. However, issues with the foot and ankle are probably connected, and the idea of regional interdependence is presented to address the overlap in the examination and treatment of musculoskeletal diseases of the foot and ankle.

While not a systematic review of the literature, this study aims to give an in-depth analysis of typical evaluations and non-pharmacologic treatment options for adult foot and ankle pain.

HURT FEET

Due to its great incidence and severe negative effects on physical performance and quality of life, foot pain has become a serious clinical and public health concern. Adults 45 years of age and older who live in the community have foot discomfort in 20–37% of cases.

At the three-year follow-up, 8.1% of older persons who had no debilitating foot pain at the baseline reported having it. People who suffer foot discomfort are significantly physically disabled, have trouble with everyday tasks and are more likely to stumble. Foot discomfort significantly lowers both overall and foot-specific quality of life.

Foot discomfort has a complex etiology, and choosing the wrong shoes may be a major contributing factor. Foot discomfort has been linked to wearing shoes that are too small or that lack stability and support (high heels, sandals, slippers). With the introduction of airbags and seat belts in recent years, a rise in the frequency of foot injuries attributable to motor vehicle trauma has been documented. The plantar impact experienced by constrained front-seat passengers may result in fractured metatarsals and ligamentous sprains. Particularly, it has been shown that motor vehicle trauma increases the incidence and severity of tarsometatarsal, talonavicular, and ankle joints.

Additionally, foot discomfort may be brought on by certain medical disorders (such as RA, gout, or osteoarthritis (OA)) or involve certain body parts (such as plantar fasciitis or Morton's neuroma). According to recent research assessing the incidence of foot symptoms in RA patients, 93.5 percent of respondents had foot pain, and 35.4% said that pain in the feet was their primary presenting symptom. 70% (14/20) of patients with acute gout flares reported foot discomfort and impairment.

When people with OA of the first metatarsophalangeal joint have severe foot discomfort, osteophytes and a higher body mass index (BMI) be modestly associated.

CLINICAL EVALUATION

Typically, the healthcare professional will note the existence of widespread foot pain during a physical examination, on interviewer-administered or self-report questionnaires, or both. Surveys and questionnaires have also been used to rate patients' self-reported foot function and impairment as well as to gauge how bad their pain is.

Subscales for evaluating pain, pain intensity, activity restriction, foot function, psychological concerns, and athletic engagement are often included in foot-specific outcomes questionnaires. In two recent systematic reviews, where one described surveys used in people with RA and the other included clinical and population-based investigations, the surveys that are presently employed were severely reviewed.

These evaluations reveal that while there are many instruments accessible, only a few numbers have undergone substantial research to determine their psychometric features (e.g. Foot Function Index, Leeds Foot Impact Scale). Particularly, there is little information on how responsiveness to change is affected by non-operative and non-pharmacologic therapies. While the majority of region-specific PROMs include the foot and ankle as well, others are tailored to a particular area or clinical group.

Despite not being foot-specific, the Lower Extremity Functional Scale (LEFS) is often utilized in clinical settings because of the previously demonstrated reliability, construct validity, and 90% confidence interval of minimum detectable change (MDC90).

The 'conventional' components of a clinical examination of the foot include a review of medical history, palpation, evaluations of sensation, range of motion, and strength, as well as specialized tests that stimulate certain tissues.

Toe deformities and skin health (dryness, sweating, perfusion) should be noticed during observation. A thorough analysis of foot examination methods and their dependability has been provided.

Static Foot Alignment and Structure

Foot structure has been measured in terms of the medial longitudinal arch's alignment and by classifying different foot kinds. The diagnostic accuracy of arch alignment (measured by sensitivity, specificity, and receiver operating characteristic, or ROC, curves) cannot be quantified objectively since the predictive usefulness of arch alignment is still debatable. Clinical (palpation-based), radiological, and foot-print-based approaches with varying degrees of validity and reliability have all been used to evaluate arch alignment. Although radiographic measurements are the "gold standard" for measuring arch alignment, they are subject to measurement mistakes because of beam location and magnification. Navicular height is commonly used in clinical practice because of its excellent concurrent validity and very simple usage.

An inexpensive jig may be used to measure the arch height index, which has good contemporaneous validity and is defined as the ratio of dorsum height to the truncated foot length. The Foot Posture Index, a six-item rating system, and a screening routine that combines clinical and radiographic approaches are examples of hybrid methods that integrate two or more examinations of arch alignment.

First metatarsophalangeal joint OA, hallux valgus, and midfoot OA have all been associated with abnormal foot anatomy, such as an elevated first ray, hypermobile first ray, and long second metatarsal, respectively. Pain and OA changes in the knee and hip have also been connected to abnormal foot anatomy. According to Gross et al., there is only a weak correlation between forefoot varus and ipsilateral hip discomfort. The likelihood of knee discomfort was 1.3 times higher in legs with low arched feet. A considerable part of the development of radiographic medial patella-femoral knee OA may be played by self-reported toe out.

Joint Motion Range

At the subtalar joint and first metatarsophalangeal joint, joint range of motion has been reliably measured using a goniometer with a one-degree resolution. In the parts that follow, the ankle is examined in further depth. To increase consistency, the rater should record the testing posture (supine, prone, or sitting), the technique utilized to stabilize the proximal joints, and whether the measurement was taken while the subject was bearing weight.

Strength Performance

Muscle strength measurements made using a hand-held dynamometer have shown to be very reliable (Intra-rater: 0.78–0.94; Inter-rater: 0.77–0.88). 3 and 1, respectively, for the intraclass correlation coefficient. To achieve inter-rater consistency, dynamometer setup and patient positioning must be standardized. Foot discomfort and diminished toe flexor strength are both independently linked to a risk of falling. People who suffer tibialis posterior tendinopathy-related foot discomfort have also been shown to have strength deficiencies.

Footwear evaluation

Examining footwear for fit (length and breadth) and design elements like the existence of a heel cup, arch support, torsional flexibility, and toe-break flexibility is recommended. It is important to take notice of any scuffing or wear patterns on the shoe's sole. The Footwear Assessment Form is a straightforward, well-structured assessment with proven face validity and reliability. To determine its applicability across cultures and clinical groups, further research could be required.

Using the Footwear Comfort Scale, one may gauge how comfortable they feel in their shoes to wear.

Analysis of Foot Motion Dynamically (including Gait Analysis)

An observational or quantitative evaluation of the foot and lower extremity mechanics while doing a weight-bearing activity is part of a dynamic assessment of foot function (e.g., walking, running, single limb squat, step down).

Because there is evidence to suggest that there is only a limited association between static and dynamic measurements of arch height and significant between-person variability, dynamic evaluations are especially pertinent in a clinical foot examination. Some writers have questioned the accuracy of observational evaluations, while others have reported adequate accuracy when employing video-based gait analysis. The studies that discovered adequate reliability included standardized video position and measuring techniques in addition to ordinal scales to determine dynamic foot alignment.

The ability to simultaneously analyze in vivo segmental foot motion together with the motion of larger proximal joints is made possible by advancements in three-dimensional motion capture technologies, which have led to improved resolution and huge capture volumes.

Dynamic Evaluation of the Distribution of Plantar Load

The plantar aspect of the foot should be examined for callus patterns and weight-bearing while doing a clinical evaluation.

In more recent years, functional activities including walking, running, stair climbing, and descending have allowed for the quantification of load distribution (plantar pressure) at the foot-floor or foot-shoe interface. Both barefoot and in-shoe pressure sensing systems are reliable. This technique was first used for those with neuropathy and diabetes who lost their sense of protection. This study will not detail how to evaluate the diabetic foot that is at risk for complications since a good overview of the topic already exists.

Elevated and prolonged plantar loading has lately been theorized to have a role in the progression of patients' self-reported foot discomfort in people. Recent studies have demonstrated higher regional plantar pressure to be present in conjunction with foot discomfort, which is consistent with this mechanical overloading idea. On the other hand, other writers contend that people with foot pain use an antalgic approach to prevent aggravating their pain. For instance, those who have 1st metatarsal-phalangeal OA may transfer their weight laterally when walking to relieve the painful area.

Similar to how RA patients with low Health Assessment Questionnaire (HAQ) ratings (greater disability, more pain) have been shown to have lower lateral forefoot loading than RA patients with high HAQ scores. Although the use of pressure measuring equipment and proper measurement techniques is rising in clinical and population-based research projects, it is still uncommon in everyday clinical practice.

Provoking examinations

The clinical examination's last phase consists of provocative tests that cause certain tissues to react. When the patient complains of discomfort when the first metatarsal-phalangeal joint is passively dorsiflexed, the Windlass test—which stretches the plantar fascia—is positive. Passive muscle length testing may be used to determine if the gastrocnemius-soleus complex or the flexor hallucis longus have restricted extensibility. Sesamoids may cause plantar discomfort and localized soreness to the touch as symptoms.

In in vivo research investigations, specialized instruments have been created to objectively measure the mobility of the first metatarsophalangeal joint and the first ray dorsal mobility; however, these devices are not often used in clinical settings.

THERAPY FOR FOOT PAIN

To provide pain relief, restore mechanics (alignment, motion, and/or load distribution), and enable the patient to resume their preferred degree of activity involvement, therapy must first address these issues. The treatment strategy should be created to address any impairments discovered during the assessment. The next subsections go into further depth on the most commonly utilized treatment methods in this clinical group, including orthoses and footwear, stretching and therapeutic exercises, manual therapy, taping, and combinational treatments.

1.Footwear and orthotics

Significant changes have been made in clinical decision-making regarding the prescription of foot orthoses during the last ten years.

There are three distinct theoretical schools of thought. The conventional strategy advocated by Root et al. concentrated on identifying foot alignment deficiencies and employed orthoses to correct static and dynamic foot alignment. The subtalar neutral position, which is operationally defined as the position in which 1) the plane passing through all five metatarsal heads is perpendicular to the calcaneal bisection and 2) the calcaneal bisection is parallel with the bisection of the lower third of the leg, was once thought to be the ideal foot alignment. Four main misalignments—rearfoot varus, rearfoot valgus, forefoot varus, and forefoot valgus—were identified based on the connection between the rearfoot and forefoot in subtalar neutral. Although the Root et almethod .'s had a significant impact on the prescription of orthoses, questions about its validity and reliability have grown. Measurement errors of 4 degrees have been recorded in studies looking at the inter-rater reliability of physicians when the foot is placed in a subtalar neutral, with weight-bearing measurements showing higher reliability. Because it might induce mistakes in the categorization of foot malalignment, measurement inaccuracy is crucial.

The validity of Root et alcategorization .'s approach has been questioned, and there aren't many normative data points available. For instance, one research (mean age: 23 years) discovered forefoot valgus in 45% of the limbs examined in women, but another group discovered forefoot varus in 87% of the limbs examined in women (mean age: 28 years). Last but not least, whereas Root et al. hypothesized a substantial correlation between static foot alignment and dynamic foot function, the predictive validity of static alignment has been disputed by objective data.

Root-based static foot alignment and dynamic foot motion did not substantially correlate in asymptomatic people.

The Tissue Stress Model has been suggested as an alternative paradigm to direct the assessment and treatment of foot diseases. This model assumes that deformation inside the elastic area of the curve will not result in symptoms and is based on an individual-specific load-deformation curve. However, damage and inflammation may arise from tissue stress in the load-deformation curve's micro failure or plastic area.

As a result, for those with foot discomfort, tissue-specific therapies such include orthoses, stretching, and targeted workouts have been suggested. Similar to this, according to the Preferred Movement Pathway idea, orthoses do not realign the bones; rather, they work by changing the input signals (forces) acting on the foot during the stance phase and the ensuing muscle activation. To prove the usefulness of these theoretical models in clinical decision-making, further proof is required.

It has been proposed that orthoses and footwear may reduce foot pain by realigning the foot, shifting plantar loads, reducing mobility, and "splinting" the troublesome joints. To reduce motion at the problematic joints in people with midfoot discomfort, steel-shanked shoes and rocker shoes are sometimes recommended. These adjustments, however, often lack acceptable visual appeal, which leads to poor adherence to therapeutic footwear. Low profile, rigid carbon graphite orthoses have lately been employed in this group as an alternative.

Braces with design elements (such as an air bladder) that provide subject-specific correction of abnormal foot mobility are offered for those with tibialis posterior tendinopathy. According to objective evidence, braces may effectively address hindfoot eversion in people with tibialis posterior tendinopathy, however, their impact on forefoot abduction may vary.

According to a recent systematic study, personalized foot orthoses should only be used sparingly to alleviate foot discomfort.However, specialist foot orthoses worked effectively for rheumatoid arthritis patients with significant pes cavus and rearfoot pain (studies show a remarkably small number needed-to-treat of only 4–5 patients for either of these specific conditions to show a benefit). For uncomfortable hallux valgus, surgery was preferable to custom orthoses, and for juvenile idiopathic arthritis, over-the-counter orthoses were just as effective.

There is no proof to back up the use of personalized orthotics for plantar heel discomfort. Custom orthoses may be costly ($300-700 each pair), and their effectiveness can vary, even though there have been relatively few negative effects associated with their usage. To anticipate whether orthoses will be effective in relieving pain, several writers have recommended using a treatment direction test. The physical examination and patient's medical history are briefly utilized to pinpoint certain actions that cause symptoms. If the patient indicates that their symptoms have improved by more than 50% with low dye tape and, if necessary, felt pads, orthoses are then recommended. Orthoses are not likely to be successful if the patient reports only little symptoms alleviation after taping.

2. Taping

Low-dye tape has been utilized in cases of plantar heel pain (plantar fasciitis) to temporarily relieve discomfort. Low-dye tape was applied for a week in recent clinical research, and the results showed that it significantly reduced "first-step" discomfort compared to sham ultrasonography.

Additionally, this study found that 28% of patients who had to tape for their condition experienced mild to severe side effects, such as discomfort from the taping being excessively tight, the onset of new pain, or an allergic response. Adverse responses could make it harder for people to tape. Taping has more recently been used to decide if a patient is a candidate for bespoke orthotics (see Treatment Direction Test in the section on Orthoses and Footwear above).

3. Stretching

Stretching is a crucial aspect of foot pain rehabilitation therapy, especially for those with heel pain. Weight-bearing and non-weight-bearing calf stretches, as well as a plantar fascia stretch carried out while the patient is sitting, are all part of the stretching regimens for heel discomfort. The patient is told to carry out each stretch at least 10 times with a 10–20 second hold, at least twice daily.

In a recent clinical investigation, tissue-specific plantar fascia stretching outperformed calf stretching in terms of pain alleviation and self-reported results after an eight-week follow-up.

4. Rehabilitation Exercise

Both targeted and generalized strength training has been recommended for people with foot discomfort and has been linked to successful results. Participation in a structured, 10–12 week eccentric strengthening program was linked to symptomatic relief and improvements in physical function in people with tibialis posterior tendinopathy. A home-based program of foot and ankle exercises together with regular foot care showed a 36 percent decrease in the risk of falls among older individuals living in communities in a recent research study. This community-based intervention includes exercises as well as orthoses, guidance on and financial assistance for footwear, a brochure on fall prevention, and regular foot care for a full year. In the section below on combination therapy, several examples of stretches and therapeutic activities are provided.

5. Manual Treatment

To treat constraints at the foot's subtalar, talocrural, and inter-tarsal joints as well as proximal joints, manual therapy uses soft tissue methods (such as trigger point release, strain counter strain), as well as joint mobilizations (hip, knee, ankle). Recent promising research suggests that soft tissue mobilization may provide temporary pain alleviation for those with heel discomfort. In comparison to a self-stretching technique, the inclusion of myofascial trigger point release offered improved short-term (single session) pain alleviation.

In the section below on combination therapy, joint mobilizations have been studied in conjunction with other modalities.

Multiple Therapies

Numerous recent studies have proposed combinational therapies to reduce pain and maximize return to activity participation, It supports the notion that functional phenotypes (sub-groups) of foot pain are defined by the presence of certain impairments (e.g., pain, loss of range of motion, poor muscle performance).

For instance, in comparison to a control group that only received physical modalities (whirlpool, ultrasound, cold packs, and electrical stimulation) and general lower extremity exercises, patients with 1st metatarsophalangeal joint pain experienced superior pain relief, restoration of range of motion, and strength with the addition of sesamoid mobilization, flexor hallucis strengthening, and gait training (calf and hamstring stretching, marble pick-up exercise). In a similar vein, patients with heel pain who received combination therapy that included joint mobilizations and stretching at a four-week follow-up showed better pain relief and self-reported physical function than those who received electro-physical agents (ultrasound and ionophoresis) and stretching.

People who have RA are especially prone to foot pain, deformities, and disability. As a result, this population is subject to aggressive preventive and monitoring strategies. Early identification of forefoot pain, diagnostic ultrasonography, and corticosteroid injection therapies for localized synovitis are strongly advised in addition to strict disease control through medical management.

There was pain alleviation and a decrease in forefoot plantar loading when stiff, full-length custom-molded orthoses were used, according to a recent systematic evaluation of the use of orthoses in rheumatoid arthritis. The maintenance of physical health and wellbeing in people with rheumatoid arthritis depends on rehabilitation programs that include components of physical exercise, strength training, and self-management in addition to foot-specific interventions.

The most important aspects of rehabilitation therapies that are helpful in the care of people with rheumatoid arthritis have been outlined in two recent studies, even though good quality data in the form of clinical trials is still rather rare. These evaluations show that even though it is commonly known that physical exercise programs may help people with RA live better lives, there is a dearth of factual information on the effects of dose and intensity. Access to multidisciplinary treatment, the use of cognitive behavioral techniques, therapeutic activity, and joint defense tactics are crucial components of effective programs.

In conclusion, the treatment of foot pain now encompasses a variety of foot-specific impairments as well as maintaining physical health via combinational therapy. There is little evidence to support the use of bespoke devices for plantar heel pain or midfoot pain, even though there is strong evidence to support thcir use in people with rheumatoid arthritis. To determine whether non-pharmacologic pain management techniques like soft-tissue mobilization and taping are effective over the long term, more research is required. Individuals with foot pain should receive self-management and community-based interventions.

AREAS FOR DEVELOPMENT IN THE EVALUATION AND TREATMENT OF FOOT PAIN

Let me underline the significance of evaluating pain processing deficiencies in those with chronic musculoskeletal pain. Pressure pain thresholds may be used to measure peripheral and central pain sensitivity in those who have foot pain. Foot pain sufferers could also engage in fear-avoidance behaviors, which might make their activity limitations and participation limits worse.

Clinical and scientific investigations are increasingly pointing to the existence of various, co-occurring deficits in people with foot discomfort. Due to the lack of large randomized clinical trials or prospective research, it will be crucial to pay close attention to study design to better understand the relationships between foot diseases and the therapies that may be used to mitigate their effects. Future research is necessary to identify functional phenotypes and the many subgroups of people who have foot discomfort. The definition of foot phenotypes is a crucial step in identifying those who are most at risk for progression and impairment, but genetic research in this area is woefully lacking. Despite being relatively novel ideas in rheumatology rehabilitation, functional phenotypes of foot disorders, including pain and impairments (such as a reduction in range of motion or poor balance), will serve as the basis for furthering our knowledge.

Ankle PAIN

Ankle discomfort has been reported by 15 percent of middle-aged and older persons in the last month, while 10 percent of older adults had radiographic ankle osteoarthritis symptoms (OA). With age, negative health outcomes include decreased physical function, balance, and gait speed as well as increased disability and fall risk are all significantly impacted by ankle discomfort and dysfunction.

While walking, the ankle joint complex—defined as the talocrural and subtalar joints—contributes between 40% and 70% of forwarding propulsion, but only 7–26% of the metabolic expenditure. Hip flexors and extensors are used more often during locomotion when ankle function is lost, increasing physiologic expenditure. The relative greater energy costs of walking experienced by older persons compared to younger adults may be explained by this change from depending on the ankle to leaning on the hip to produce forward propulsion during gait.

Additionally, studies comparing high- and low-performing older persons who live in the community indicate that those with superior ankle function have greater levels of mobility and functional status than those with poor ankle function.

The inability to reach 10° of dorsiflexion during the stride, or equinus, is a frequent reason for ankle dysfunction. Equinus, which is characterized by impaired ankle mobility and function, may be brought on by the gastrocnemius and/or soleus muscles becoming stiffer.

Aging and a lack of exercise, which tend to reduce flexibility, are two major risk factors for equinus.

Ankle osteoarthritis may also contribute to poor ankle function (OA). A 10% prevalence of ankle OA is seen in those over the age of 65. Ankle OA is mostly caused by post-traumatic ankle OA, which accounts for around 4 out of 5 cases. Post-traumatic OA is most often caused by fracture events, primarily malleolar or tibial plafond fractures, which are frequently caused by auto accidents.

Ligamentous injuries accounted for 16 percent of patients. Less than 10% of ankle OA patients include primary OA.

The emphasis of this section will be on the diagnostic and non-pharmacologic treatment methods of chronic ankle dysfunction, such as that which comes from equinus or arthritis, even though acute ankle injuries are one of the most common physical injuries that cause ER visits.

CLINICAL EVALUATION

Measures of patient-reported outcomes (PROMs)

Patients' opinions of their health and function are evaluated using patient-reported outcome measures (PROMs). Ankle PROMs often include questions on the quality of life, mobility, pain, and function. They are used as a measuring tool to evaluate the impact of illness or damage on function, and the impact of therapy, and to identify potential substantive changes on an individual basis.

Numerous surveys have been used in outcome-based studies with little to no evidence to support their utility, according to a systematic review analyzing PROMs in ankle function, pain, and health. They discovered 49 distinct rating scales for ankle-specific instruments in their research, although many PROMs lacked construct and content validity as well as reliability and proof of responsiveness. Twelve ankle-related PROMs were shown to exhibit construct validity, reliability, and content validity in recent systematic studies.

However, it is significant to highlight that only two PROMs discuss the importance of footwear choice and orthotics, and the majority of instruments do not contain questions that address the psychological aspect of ankle pain and dysfunction.

When using PROMs, care should be given to verify that the outcome measure of interest has been validated in the population and addresses the proper content domains of the research. This is because PROMs are validated in particular populations.

Five PROMs evaluate ankle ligament or acute injuries, four PROMs support the use of generalized orthopedic and pathological conditions of the foot and ankle, two PROMs assess chronic ankle instability, and one PROM evaluates ankle joint complex fractures, juvenile arthritis, lower extremity function, and ankle osteoarthritis among the common conditions that affect the ankle (OA).

The value of computerized adaptive testing, which may shorten assessment times and enhance the comparability of PROM outcomes across studies, should be addressed in future guidelines for ankle PROMs.

Ankle-foot Alignment

Ankle arthritis, discomfort, and disability are strongly influenced by foot-ankle alignment, which has been measured as the calcaneal stance position at rest (RCSP).

A composite measure that combines the malleolar valgus index (VMI), the rearfoot alignment view, and the long leg calcaneal axial view has shown great accuracy (r = 0.814) in the evaluation of RCSP. VMI is a static measurement of the plantar foot obtained using a flatbed computer scan. VMI is determined by dividing the distance from the transmalleolar width's center to the foot bisection's heel by 100. Although various cut-off angles are utilized, rearfoot alignment in terms of rearfoot varus/valgus is covered in the section on static structure and alignment of the foot.

A radiographic method called the long leg calcaneal axial view gives a view of the subtalar space and the alignment of the calcaneus with the tibia. However, integrating these tests into clinical settings may be difficult since they need a lot of setup and equipment.

Joint Motion Range

When evaluating ankle range of motion, measurement methods differ greatly. The amount of weight bearing, the degree of knee flexion, and whether or not ankle ROM was evaluated actively or passively are important factors to take into account.

In comparison to non-weight bearing, ROM is often greater during weight bearing. The Norkin and White technique, in which participants position one foot in front of the other and bend the knee of the front leg in a squat as low as they can while keeping their body straight and their heels on the ground, or in a weight-bearing lunge, is an example of a weight-bearing measure. Researchers challenge the external validity of ROM assessed in the non-weight bearing position since the ankle generally works in partial or full weight bearing during movement, and studies often report both a weight-bearing and non-weight bearing assessment of ankle ROM.

While passive measurements of ROM use a device or a clinician moving the ankle joint through the range of motion, active measures of ROM require the subject to move the ankle joint. Lack of uniformity among examiners is a typical issue with ankle ROM measurements.

While inter-rater goniometric measures show low to moderate (0.5-0.8) reliability, independent of method or rater expertise, intra-rater reliabilities and intraclass correlation coefficients (ICCs) is often more than 0.9 regardless of the technique. Since the range of normal ankle dorsiflexion extends from 0° to 13.1° and the range of normal ankle ROM is 50° to 75°, inter-rater readings may have a variance of 7° between testers.

There is a need for the employment of standardized, valid, and reliable approaches to evaluate ankle ROM given the vast range of goniometer values and the often poor

reproducibility of these measurements.

Muscular Power

Manual muscle testing is a common method for evaluating muscle strength (MMT). MMT does not define strength; instead, it evaluates strength using an ordinal grading system.

To measure the strength of the plantar flexors, MMT at the ankle joint includes heel rises, which the subject is instructed to repeat as many as feasible. Participants are regarded as having better strength if they finish more repetitions. Although there are other ranking methods, MMT may also be evaluated by how well the muscle can withstand the power of the examiner. The degree of resistance is ranked ordinally as follows: 5 = normal, 4 = excellent, 3 = fair, 2 = poor, 1 = trace, 0 = zero or absence of contraction.

Despite the grading system's subjectivity, it may be made very trustworthy by trained, experienced assessors (ICCs greater than 0.93). Studies of examiner-assessed MMT also indicate that dorsiflexion has a significant degree of intraclass correlation coefficient (ICC) variability (range 0.58–0.92) and that plantarflexion muscle weakness is underappreciated in terms of frequency and severity.

Instrumented measurements of ankle strength and power include dynamometer measurements of torque and power during dorsiflexion and plantarflexion.

Because patient-initiated intra-rater and inter-rater ICCs are 0.95 or higher, and clinician-initiated ICCs are often less than 0.80, the testing method used with a hand-held dynamometer may have an impact on reliability. The computerized dynamometry ICCs vary from 0.84 to 0.99 for the maximum peak torque, average peak torque, power, and work. For average peak torque, power and work, and maximum torque, Capranica et al. observed lower ICCs, ranging from 0.29 to 0.80, although their speeds were greater at 90°/second, as opposed to 60°/second.

It is important to remember that the patient must be mechanically grounded by having their trunk fastened and their proximal segment stabilized. Assessment of muscle strength is especially important for those with ankle OA since they have significantly weaker ankle plantarflexion muscles than those on the opposite side.

Proprioception

Proprioception, or the body's capacity to recognize its motion and position, is a crucial aspect of balance and injury avoidance.

Proprioception may be evaluated using two major methods: 1) Joint angle reproduction, and 2) threshold of detecting passive motion (JAR). Joint kinesthesia and the body's capacity to recognize passive motion are assessed by TDPM testing. The ankle joint is moved slowly—0.4°/s on a computerized dynamometer—and the amount of sagittal or frontal plane movement that occurs before the subject notices the motion is recorded. The kinesthetic awareness is worse the more joint movement there is before it is noticed.

In JAR testing, the ankle joint is passively or actively adjusted at a predetermined target angle, and the subject is instructed to reproduce the angle. Both a relative angle, which represents an offshoot (positive angle) or an undershoot (negative angle) and an absolute angle, which represents the total number of degrees from the goal angle, are recorded for the number of degrees away from the target angle.

While TDPM and JAR are standard proprioception measurements at the knee joint, further study is needed to understand how joint proprioception influences ankle joint function and raises the risk of injury and falls at the ankle joint.

Dynamic Evaluation of Ankle Movement (including Gait Analysis)

It is possible to use gait analysis (three-dimensional motion capture or two-dimensional video) to assess a person's walking pattern or other actions like cutting or leaping.

Joint moments may be calculated by combining motion capture with a force plate for a kinetic (e.g., force data) evaluation. Motion capture gives a kinematic (e.g., joint angles, displacements) assessment. Even though these technologies might be expensive, they provide a more accurate way to quantify movement (motion capture has an ICC of > 0.75 compared to observational gait analysis's ICC of 0.75). Furthermore, modern technology now makes it possible to quantify joint mobility in vivo with extreme accuracy and precision using bi-planar x-ray fluoroscopy.

Instrumented and non-instrumented balance tests, especially single-leg exercises, are often used to assess balance deficiencies. The measurement of the center of pressure displacement while calm standing is often used in sway pattern analysis. The Star Excursion Balance Test figure-of-eight hop, side hop, up-down hop, single-leg hop for distance, and agility hop test are other typical functional evaluations.

Provoking examinations

There are various techniques available to determine ankle laxity because of the potential danger of ankle OA and the significant residual impairment that follows acute ankle trauma. To evaluate the strength of the lateral ligaments, common tests include the anterior drawer and talar tilt test. The external rotation (Kleiger) or squeezing tests are suggested when tibiofibular syndesmosis damage is suspected. A strong index of suspicion is necessary since syndesmotic tests are known for their high specificity but relatively poor sensitivity.

In recent years, it has become clear that ankle impingement may cause lateral-sided ankle discomfort, especially in those who have already had an ankle sprain. Despite the recent publication of a provocative test for anterolateral impingement, nothing is known about its sensitivity and specificity as of the time of this study. An osteochondral lesion of the talar dome may be the cause of persistent deep, throbbing ankle discomfort on the lateral side. Tibialis posterior tendinopathy should be included in the differential diagnosis of medial-sided ankle pain because deltoid ligament injuries are uncommon.

Achilles tendinopathy, posterior impingement, and retro-calcaneal bursitis are three conditions that can cause pain on the ankle's backside.

HOW TO HEAL ANKLE PAIN

Similar to how foot pain is treated, the main goals of therapy for people with ankle pain are to lessen symptoms, improve mechanics (such as alignment, mobility, and/or load distribution), and get the patient back to the level of activity involvement they had hoped for.

The treatment strategy should be created to address any impairments discovered during the assessment. Stretching, manual therapy, therapeutic exercises, footwear modification, and orthoses are the most commonly employed treatment modalities in this clinical group and are covered in more depth in the following subsections.

1.Stretching

Adults should engage in at least 30 minutes of moderate-intensity aerobic activity five days a week, along with two days of muscle-building exercises and two to three days of flexibility training.

These recommendations state that stretches should be performed two to four times for a total of 60 seconds every stretch, held for 10 to 30 seconds until the point of tightness or mild pain. A meta-analysis suggests that the clinical significance of stretching in asymptomatic younger adults is unknown. Studies evaluating the effects of stretching the muscles of the ankle joint complex (e.g., gastrocnemius, soleus, anterior tibialis) have shown mixed results, with some studies suggesting ankle ROM can be enhanced and others noting no significant gains.

Studies, however, reveal that older persons may dramatically increase their ankle ROM and that long stretch durations for each repetition—for example, holding each stretch for 60 seconds as opposed to 15 or 30—are more likely to do so. Passive stiffness also improves together with the increase in anklc ROM in older persons, albeit not always with an increase in gait speed.

2. Manual Treatment

For those with limited active ankle dorsiflexion, studies on the short-term effects of a single intervention of trigger point massage plus joint mobilization or manipulation revealed increases of about 5 degrees. High-velocity thrust manipulations, however, have not significantly improved ankle range of motion (ROM) or muscle activation in people with lateral ankle sprains. There aren't many studies looking at manual therapies at the ankle joint, thus further study is required to see how they affect physical function and mobility in addition to the function of the ankle joint.

3. Rehabilitation Exercise

Isometric exercises in plantarflexion, dorsiflexion, inversion, and eversion against an immovable object, as well as dynamic resistance exercises using ankle weights, surgical tubing, or resistance bands, are often used to strengthen the ankle. For those with Achilles tendinopathy, high resistance eccentric exercise is particularly advised.

Exercises involving the foot and ankle movements have also produced effective interventions. According to Hartman et al., compared to a general exercise program without foot gymnastics, a general exercise program with foot gymnastics enhanced foot and ankle function. The foot gymnastics consisted of three parts: (1) a 2-min warm-up activity that included heel-to-toe lifts and walking on both heels and toes; (2) 4-min foot exercises that involved spreading and moving the toes; catching small items (like marbles); and (3) 4-min static ankle stretching.

Participants in this group demonstrated gains in muscular strength and gait speed above those who just participated in the generalist exercise program after 12 weeks of exercise and foot gymnastics. Similar to this, Benedetti et al. found that compared to general workouts, individuals in an exercise program focusing on flexibility and strength growth improved their strength, range of motion, and posture.

The flexibility and strength of the ankles have both improved with therapeutic activities like Tai Chi.

According to a recent meta-analysis, Tai Chi exercise strengthens the ankle flexor and extensor muscles in older adults. Long-term Tai Chi practitioners also have better ankle proprioception than long-term swimmers, runners, and sedentary people. A 16-week study, however, was unable to demonstrate how practicing Tai Chi improved ankle proprioception. Together, these findings imply that improvements in mobility brought about by exercise programs can increase ankle functionality; however, more research is required to pinpoint precise elements relating to dosage, intensity, and patient choice to achieve the best results.

4, Footwear adaptations and orthoses

Orthotics and footwear alterations have both been used to treat people with ankle discomfort. People with impaired ankle ROM and function have been treated using rocker-style shoes in particular. When sagittal plane ankle mobility is limited, adding rocker bottoms to the shoe may help with ankle motion and increase forward propulsion.

The rocker sole shoe's main functions are to encourage heel-toe gait, minimize shoe flexing to regain ankle function and unload pressure points on the foot. People with ankle problems often use heel-toe or negative heel rockers out of the several types of rocker soles. Using a negative rocker or acting within the available ankle ROM, heel-toe, or negative rocker soles, the pitch of the rocker in rocker-style shoes should be adapted to the particular ankle position (such as an ankle stuck in dorsiflexion). People with impaired balance or Achilles tendon contracture should not use the negative type rocking chair.

Additionally, employing heel lifts with shoes that have a little rocker might result in a negative rocker sole and encourage a heel-toe gait. Rocker-style shoes may be worn by themselves or in conjunction with a cushioned heel to help improve gait and ankle range of motion in individuals with arthritis. Although identifying the ideal rocker position might be difficult, the success of the therapy can be assessed using an in-sole plantar pressure device.

Those with ankle discomfort and dysfunction may also benefit from orthoses on their own.

According to studies comparing a rigid hindfoot orthosis, an articulated hindfoot orthosis, and a custom ankle-foot orthosis for people with subtalar and ankle OA, the rigid hindfoot orthosis significantly restricted ankle motion while allowing enough forefoot movement under different walking circumstances (e.g., on a ramp). People with ankle discomfort brought on by subtalar or ankle OA may find this therapy helpful because of the regulated motion the stiff hindfoot orthosis provides.

Men, older persons, and those with less pain benefit more from an orthotic intervention for ankle dysfunction, which implies that other therapies are required to close the treatment gap for other categories. The capacity of the ankle to produce force during push-off during walking may be compromised by extended use of devices that limit motion, even while they provide significant pain relief. Prolonged usage may also lead to loss of joint mobility and muscle strength. As a result, low-profile, lightweight ankle-foot orthoses with elastic recoil are becoming more and more popular.

AREAS FOR DEVELOPMENT IN THE EVALUATION AND TREATMENT OF ANKLE PAIN

Following acute ankle injuries, residual ankle impairment and dysfunction are frequent, which may cause chronic ankle discomfort, mobility restrictions, and a "feeling of giving way" in addition to other symptoms. A growing number of people are becoming aware that osteochondral injuries and persistent ankle instability may act as risk factors for developing ankle discomfort and OA.

As a result, during evaluation, early detection and a high index of suspicion are required. Deficits in ankle range of motion (ROM), strength, and balance are known to increase the risk of falling in older persons. With the ultimate objective of getting the patient back to their desired level of activity participation and avoiding re-injury, intervention measures should not only concentrate on pain treatment and gait retraining, but also fall avoidance and neuromuscular training.

Chapter 4

Central Command: The Hips and Pelvis

The pelvic girdle, the skeletal structure that connects the axial skeleton to the lower limbs, is made up of the left and right hip bones, also known as innominate bones or pelvic bones.

There are three primary articulations on the hip bones:

• The sacrum and sacroiliac joint articulate.

• The pubic symphysis is the joint where the left and right hip bones meet.

• Articulation of the hip joint with the femoral head.

Hip dislocation

Ilium, pubis, and ischium are the three components that make up the hip bone. The triradiate cartilage divides these portions before puberty, and fusion doesn't start until a person is between the ages of 15 and 17.

The acetabulum, literally "vinegar cup" in Latin, is a cup-shaped socket formed by the ilium, pubis, and ischium. The hip joint is created by the head of the femur articulating with the acetabulum.

Female reproductive organs

The bladder, lower parts of the ureters, and the urethra are urologic viscera. The pubic bone and symphysis are directly superior and posterior to the bladder, which is situated anterior to the uterus. The bladder is joined to the pubic symphysis anteriorly by fibrous ligaments. From the bladder to the umbilicus, the urachus runs. The ureters start at the renal calyxes and are located on the anterior side of the psoas muscle, just lateral to the ovarian vessels and vena cava.

The ureters then cross the pelvic brim over the common iliac arteries and enter the pelvis along the lateral pelvic sidewall. The ureters subsequently enter the trigone area of the bladder (the triangular portion of the bladder base).

The uterus, fallopian tubes, and ovaries are included in the group of gynecologic viscera. Between the bladder and rectosigmoid colon, these structures are located in the middle. The fundus (upper section), lower segment, and cervix are the three segments of the uterus.

Concerning the vagina and cervix, the uterus is most often anteverted (meaning the cervix angles forward) and anteflexed (meaning the body of the uterus bends forward), which causes the uterus to lay just above the bladder. A pregnant woman's uterus grows to 20 times its normal size and weight at term. The uterus shrinks and atrophies after menopause compared to a woman of reproductive age. The cervix, which divides the uterus from and extends into the vagina, is thick and fibromuscular.

At the level of the ischial spines and fifth sacral vertebra, where the pelvic diaphragm muscles are hung above the cervix and upper vagina (S5). The fallopian tubes are bilateral structures that extend 10 to 14 cm from the superior-lateral part of the uterus. They are typically less than 1 cm thick. The infundibulum is the distal end of the fallopian tube, and finger-like extensions freely protrude from this end of the tube. Close to the iliac arteries and ureters, the ovaries are located in the ovarian fossa of the peritoneum.

Numerous ligamentous structures are projected from the uterus.

The fibrous and muscular circular ligaments are situated in the uterus right in front of the fallopian tubes. The circular ligaments go through the internal inguinal ring, via the external iliac vessels, and then into the labia majora. The peritoneum folds over the round ligaments to form the wide ligament. The uterus receives very modest support from the large and rounded ligaments. The rounded ligament directs the ovaries into the proper position during the development of a female fetus.

The round ligament helps to draw the bladder anteriorly, above the uterus, as people age. The vesicouterine fossa (anterior to the uterus) and the rectouterine fossa are formed by the division of the pelvic cavity by the wide ligament, a folded sheet of peritoneum covering the uterus, uterine tubes, and ovaries (posterior to the uterus). The cardinal ligament, which links laterally from the cervix to the endopelvic fascia, serves as the primary support for the uterus and cervix (which is attached to the pelvic bone).

The uterosacral ligaments start at the superior-posterior part of the cervix and go bilaterally across the rectum before attaching to the sacral vertebrae (first through fifth) to support the cervix in various ways.

The rectum, which is located along the curve of the sacrum posterior to the uterus, is the section of the gastrointestinal viscera in the pelvis. Pathologic diseases including endometriosis, malignancy, or pelvic adhesions may reside in the posterior cul-de-sac between the uterus and rectum.

Muscles, ligaments, arteries, and nerves work together to provide dynamic support for the whole viscera that are contained in the pelvis. There are three external entrances to the pelvis: the urethra (bladder), vagina (uterus), and anus (rectum). These devices may maintain bladder and bowel continence while also allowing for voluntary urination and defecation. Significant stresses such as persistent intraabdominal pressure and vaginal labor and delivery may be applied to the dynamic support (e.g., chronic constipation or long-term heavy lifting).

Skeletal female pelvis

The bilateral innominate bones (the ilium, ischium, and pubis bones), the sacrum, and the coccyx make up the bony pelvis, which is shaped like a ring. The femoral head articulates with the innominate's acetabulum (hip bone). The pelvis of a man and a woman are different. The female pelvis and explaining the numerous pelvic forms are the main topics of this article. Gynecoid, anthropoid, android, or platypelloid shapes are possible for the bony pelvis.

A gynecoid pelvic form, which has a round inlet, straight sidewalls, an average prominence of ischial spines, well-rounded sacrosciatic notches, a well-curved sacrum, and roomy subpubic arches (> 90-degree angle), is the typical pelvic shape for women. It accounts for 50% of all females. The gynecoid form is roomier and is thus perfect for childbirth. Women make up about 30% of the population and have an android form with a triangle intake (in which arrest of descent during labor and delivery is common). The male pelvis often has the android form.

The fetal head engages in the occiput posterior position during birth in 20% of women due to their oval anthropoid form (occipitoanterior is the desirable position). A flattened gynecoid form known as the platypelloid is seen in around 3 percent of females. The traditional male pelvis is intrinsically more stable than the female pelvis due to its bony nature; the female pelvis' form encourages movement during labor and delivery.

Genital ligaments

The pelvic ligaments range in structure and function from dense connective tissues with high structural support to smooth, musculoskeletal, fibrous, and areolar tissues with little structural support. The larger and lesser sciatic foramina, which enable transit of neurovascular systems from inside the pelvis to the lower extremities and genital area, are formed by the sacrospinous and sacrotuberous ligaments. These two thick ligaments help keep the pelvic joints stable, coupled with the anterior longitudinal ligament of the sacrum.

The gynecologic viscera are previously mentioned in connection to the ligaments extending from uterine tissues.

The pelvic muscles

The "pelvic diaphragm" and the pelvic wall muscles are among the muscles of the pelvis.

The levator ani (puborectalis, pubococcygeus, and iliococcygeus) and coccygeus are the muscles of the pelvic diaphragm. The pelvic viscera are supported by these muscles, which act as their core and primary support system.

These muscles originate in the lateral pelvic wall, go downhill and medially, and then merge in the center and behind. The urethra, vagina, and anus may pass through the levator hiatus, which is an opening inside these muscles on the anterior side. To sustain the abdominopelvic contents against intraabdominal stresses, the type I (slow twitch) fibers of the pelvic diaphragm muscles typically maintain a consistent tone. These muscles avoid persistent tension on the ligaments and fascia of the pelvis by doing this.

The pelvic diaphragm's type II (rapid twitch) fibers allow for swift contractions to give support in response to transient increases in abdominal pressure (e.g., when coughing, sneezing, or jumping). These muscles raise superiorly as they contract (voluntarily or involuntarily), flexing the anorectal canal to allow for fecal continence and voluntary bladder control. Only momentarily and sporadically can these muscles relax to enable the anorectal canal to straighten for fecal emptying, bladder emptying, and fetal head direction during birth.

The S2 to S4 nerve root innervates the hybrid (smooth and striated muscle tissue) pelvic muscles. The perineal membrane and perineal body support the pelvic diaphragm and are inferior to (more superficial than) the pelvic diaphragm muscles.

The piriformis and obturator internus are two muscles on the pelvic wall. The inferior, lateral, and posterior pelvic walls are partly covered by the striated fasciae of these muscles. The piriformis muscle arises from the anterior-lateral surface of the sacrum and fills a portion of the posterior-lateral pelvic wall.

By passing through the greater sciatic foramen and attaching to the greater trochanter of the femur, the piriformis emerges from the pelvic cavity. The obturator internus, which develops from the ilium, ischium, and obturator membrane inside the pelvis, occupies a portion of the sidewalls of the pelvis. The lesser sciatic foramen is where the obturator internus exits the pelvis before turning and continuing to insert onto the greater trochanter of the femur. The arcus tendinous levator ani (ATLA), which serves as the place of origin for some of the levator ani muscles, is a thickening of fascia on the surface of the obturator internus.

The arcus tendinous fascia pelvis (ATFP), another fascial thickening, travels from the inner pubic bones to the ischial spines and offers a lateral point of attachment for the anterior vaginal wall. It covers the medial side of the levator ani and obturator internus muscles.

The pelvic nerves

Supradiaphragmatic and infra diaphragmatic parts of the pelvis are innervated. Control of the bladder, uterus, and rectum is part of the supradiaphragmatic system (including autonomic nervous system regulation of urethral and anal sphincter tone).

As smooth muscle sphincters constrict in response to sympathetic input, the bladder and rectum may typically hold urine and feces, respectively. The bulk of the sympathetic innervation comes from the hypogastric plexuses and the sacral sympathetic trunk (minority). The bladder outlet, urethral sphincters, and anal sphincters all relax as a result of parasympathetic input, allowing urine and feces to be released. The sacral spinal nerves are the source of parasympathetic innervation. During surgery or labor and delivery, the autonomic nerve structures may be harmed (pelvic or spinal).

The pudendal nerve and its branches provide practically all of the somatic innervation of the infra diaphragmatic motor system. The S2 to S4 nerve roots give birth to the pudendal nerve. The internal pudendal artery and vein accompany it as it passes through the pudendal canal (along the ischiorectal fossa) after exiting the pelvis through the greater sciatic foramen, running posterior to the sacrospinous ligament, and then entering the pelvis again through the lesser sciatic foramen. Pudendal nerve compression may occur in the area between the sacrospinous and sacrotuberous ligaments.

The striated muscles of the urethra and anus are innervated by the pudendal nerve, together with the motor innervation of the urogenital diaphragm and cutaneous innervation of the external genitalia. The inferior rectal branch, the perineal branch, and the anterior (clitoral) branch are the three branches of the pudendal nerve. The levator ani nerve, which supplies the pelvic diaphragm muscles, passes along the top of the coccygeus muscle, immediately medial to the ischial spine.

Pelvic and Hip Anatomical Relationships

The main mechanism for transmitting weight and forces from the trunk and upper limbs to the lower limbs is the bony pelvis. Additionally, it gives the muscles of the trunk and lowers extremities somewhere to connect, which may lessen discomfort and dysfunction in the hip and pelvis. It is useful in the therapeutic therapy and proper referral of patients with pelvic and hip discomfort or other problems to have an understanding of the muscles that connect to the pelvis, hip joint, and lower extremities.

The quadriceps femoris, pectineus, iliopsoas, and sartorius muscles are located in the anterior fascial compartment of the thigh. The sartorius originates from the anterior superior iliac spine (ASIS), crosses the hip, and continues distally until joining the medial tibial surface. The rectus femoris originates from the anterior inferior iliac spine (AIIS) and the ilium just above the acetabulum. It subsequently inserts on the patella and converges with other quadriceps tendons to insert on the tibial tuberosity. The origin of the iliacus, which joins the psoas to create the iliopsoas, originates in the iliac fossa.

The iliopsoas then goes under the inguinal ligament and connects to the lesser trochanter of the femur. The pectineus, which likewise inserts on the lesser trochanter of the femur, originates from the pectin pubis. The gracilis, obturator internus, adductor longus, brevis, and adductor component of the adductor Magnus (pubofemoral section) muscles are located in the medial compartment of the thigh. The gracilis emerges and inserts into the medial tibia from the inferior pubic ramus and ramus of the ischium. The obturator internus arises from the pubic and ischial rami, the obturator membrane, and inserts into the greater trochanter of the femur. The adductors originate from the pubic ramus and ischial tuberosity. The biceps femoris, semitendinosus, semimembranosus, and hamstring component of the adductor Magnus (ischiocondylar section) muscles are located in the posterior compartment of the thigh. All of these muscles have their origins in the ischial tuberosity. The semitendinosus attaches to the medial tibia, the semimembranosus to the medial tibial condyle, and the hamstring component of the adductor Magnus to the adductor tubercle of the femur.

The biceps femoris inserts into the head of the fibula. As they go from the pelvis to the superior femur and trochanter, the gluteus medius and minimus, piriformis, gemellus superior and inferior, obturator internus, and quadratus femoris are also involved.

It is important to take into account the physiological variations between the muscular systems of men and women when evaluating the muscular connections between the hip and pelvis. Males see an increase in lean muscle mass when they enter adolescence, whereas females experience an increase in fat deposits but not in lean muscle mass. 12 During puberty, this fat deposition causes the growth of female breasts and the broadening of the hips. Girls have around 75% of the strength of males by the middle of adolescence. In addition, compared to males, women have a larger percentage of type I fibers (slow twitch). A greater risk of certain injuries in girls and women has been linked to variations in muscle function. Unlike boys and men who contract the hamstrings, female athletes exhibit contraction of the quadriceps with anterior tibial disturbance.

Girls and women are also less able to stabilize the knee in an anterior-posterior plane and less able to tighten muscles surrounding the knee when heavy internal rotation is happening. Poor hip-knee control during landing after a jump is one of the characteristics linked to higher risks of anterior cruciate ligament injuries. Differences in quadriceps activity may be related to patellofemoral discomfort (timing, intensity, torque production).

The neurological connections between the hip and pelvis are the last factor to take into account.

From the lower trunk and pelvis, many nerves branch out to the hip, thigh, and perineal tissues. The lateral psoas muscle is where the ilioinguinal, iliohypogastric, lateral femoral cutaneous, and femoral nerves leave the body. The belly of the psoas houses the genitofemoral nerve. The obturator nerve leaves the psoas muscle medially and enters the obturator foramen. Each of these nerves is susceptible to compression and irritation due to pregnancy-related structural changes, iliopsoas involvement, and tightness.

Additionally, the piriformis muscle is where the sciatic nerve crosses superiorly, through, or inferiorly; piriformis tension or spasm may cause sciatic nerve discomfort. Paresthesia of the lateral thigh may come from compression of the lateral femoral cutaneous nerve, which can happen when the inguinal ligament and abdomen are compressed or while wearing tight clothes. Concerning particular diseases, this chapter goes into further detail on the neural connections between the hip and pelvis.

Conclusion

It can seem that all three stories can provide the same explanation.

A puzzling phenomenon involving pain, since all three stories

One's attitudes and beliefs affect how thcy feel throughout their

experience of agony. In actuality, the many cognitive models

These pain descriptions imply that they may be sufficient.

Factors that assist almost any pain causes phenomenon. However, it's also conceivable that these

Accounts suggest differences when they are empirical significant. It seems at the very least that whether a discomfort

Scientists consider pain in the same ways that Hall, Pitcher, or Douglas do. would affect the questions one is trying to answer. responses to. For instance, whether one considers chronic

In terms of pain (in the absence of any physical harm), a perceptual system's reporting of deceptive information, or as an unusual manner of feeling a typical experience will result into various prejudices and research objectives. In the latter scenario, one may think about how different antidepressants affect chronic pain. In the first scenario, one may look for additional in-depth information about the physical harm technique for recognizing potential causes of the "misfire."

While both research agendas may eventually coexist add to our understanding of how to cure persistent pain,,is plausible to anticipate the most consistent flow of clinical advancements once we get a reliable model of the processes of processing that underlie pain.

Should philosophers then conclude that the ultimate

Is the best way to settle the aforementioned argument to submit it to psychologists?

If there are genuine factual discrepancies between the opposing methods to comprehend pain from a perceptual standpoint, then

It should ultimately be up to those doing the empirical research.

To determine which viewpoint is most consistent with the strongest mental model. Maybe this much is obvious: one method proceed with the philosophical discussion of the there is a connection between pain and perception.

Experts to share their opinions on theMfoundational cognitive paradigms. They could also provide their perspectives on whether the different connections suggested by

There is significant empirical value in philosophers.

It's not, however, appropriate to ask empirical scientists for their opinion.

Neither giving up the intellectual endeavor nor dismissing the

Folk perception of pain is that it is completely meaningless or irrelevant.

Nor is it true that philosophical inquiry into pain has advanced to

it's sizing. Instead, it is only to acknowledge that the philosophical analysis of pain and associated research on

Greater clarity in perception and feeling

Understanding of how psychologists interpret such ideas

As "perception," "feeling," and what they consider to be pain ideal models.

In the end, our present "folk" ideas of pain perception, associated psychological factors, and

It is impossible to separate notions from one another. a bigger either one's comprehension may progress our comprehension of the other.